PREHAB BEFORE POSTPARTUM

A Perinatal Depression And Anxiety Guide For A Happier Postpartum

DR. RAUSHANAH HUD-ALEEM

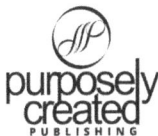

purposely created
PUBLISHING

PREHAB BEFORE POSTPARTUM
Published by Purposely Created Publishing Group™
Copyright © 2019 Raushanah Hud-Aleem

All rights reserved.

Printed in the United States of America

ISBN: 978-1-64484-032-0

DEDICATION

I first want to thank the Almighty Creator for the count-less blessings, being merciful, and for allowing me to serve. I would also like to thank my parents for the love and sacrifices they made to afford my siblings and I op-portunities for success. Thank you to my father and un-cle for engaging in entrepreneurship and modeling the importance of creating wealth for the longevity of our legacy and our community. To my mother-in-law, all my aunts, cousins, play cousins, and friends, thank you for your prayers and support. To my husband, my best friend, my confidant, thank you for your love, patience, and support. I could not have done this without you. You are a wonderful father. I feel blessed that you are my life partner. I want to thank my four beautiful daughters: Layla, Surayyah, Niyyah, and Minnah for your inspira-tion. I want to thank all my siblings for being supportive. Thank you to my sister, Dr. Zarinah, for pushing me and being an example for her big sister. Thank you, Dr. Drai and my fellow medical moguls for your support. Thank you, Dr. Drai for your mentorship and helping me begin this journey of independence and service. Finally, thank you to all the women who have dealt with perinatal depression and anxiety for being an inspiration to me, and thanks to all those health professionals who are on the front line trying to improve mental wellness and increase knowledge and understanding, while decreasing stigma.

EPIGRAPH

"We wear the mask that grins and lies,
It hides our cheeks and shades our eyes, —
This debt we pay to human guile;
With torn and bleeding hearts we smile,
And mouth with myriad subtleties.

Why should the world be over-wise,
In counting all our tears and sighs?
Nay, let them only see us, while
 We wear the mask."

Paul Laurence Dunbar (Dunbar, 1913)

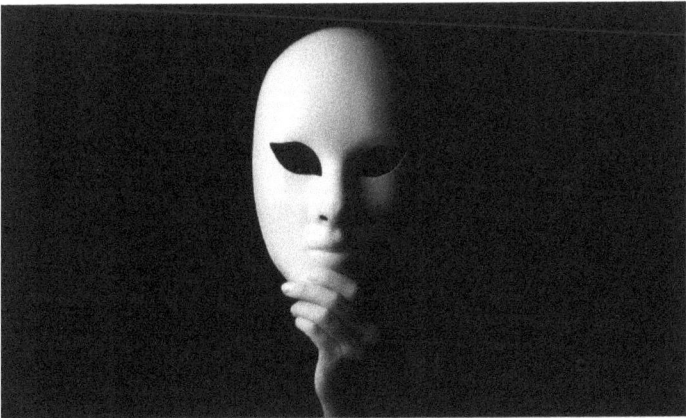

TABLE OF CONTENTS

INTRODUCTION

I am the daughter of two mental health professionals who worked with underserved children and their families. Education and family are some of the core values they instilled into my siblings and me. These values led me to becoming a honor roll student athlete in high school, magna cum laude college graduate, and double board-certified adult, child, and adolescent psychiatrist with over 17,000 encounters serving underserved children and families.

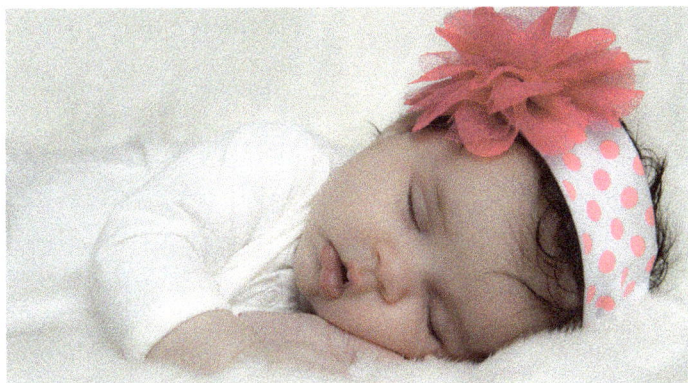

As many young girls do, I played house with my sisters and dreamed of one day getting married and having children. I thought it would be just as easy as it appeared on television. So when my husband and I decided to start a family, I anticipated that I would get pregnant right away; the pregnancy would be blissful, and labor quick and uneventful. After delivery, I thought nursing would be easy, I would make homemade baby food and be the perfect wife and perfect mother. This was far from my reality.

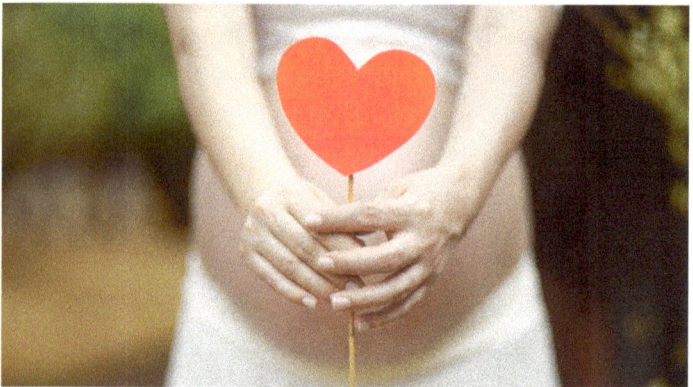

I want to share my story and take off my mask. I am the mother of four beautiful daughters, and I have suffered from postpartum depression and anxiety with every pregnancy. Each pregnancy was different. However, the first and last one was the most challenging.

My first pregnancy was uneventful until delivery. Everything I thought I learned from the pregnancy classes, reading books, talking to other mothers, etc., went right out the window. I was in labor for a very long time and the doctor was contemplating a C-section. Instead, my delivery wound up being assisted via forceps, a traumatic event for both me and my baby. Right after delivery, I immediately tried breastfeeding, literally while still on the delivery bed, and it was one of the most difficult and painful experiences. This beautiful fragile little creature had the jaws of life. How could something so natural be so painful? How can a medical school graduate not be able to manage something so "elementary" as breastfeeding, I thought. I was determined to get it, however. After continued difficulty with breastfeeding, I requested assistance from a lactation specialist while in the hospital with little success.

I was discharged from the hospital and continued to struggle with getting the baby to latch. At the same time, I experienced swelling, sore nipples, headaches, and extreme fatigue. I went to see my OB about two or three days after discharge, and she immediately sent me to the emergency room to be admitted to the ICU. My blood pressure was 210/105. I was ultimately diagnosed with postpartum pre-eclampsia, a rare condition that occurs when a woman has high blood pressure and excess protein in her urine soon after childbirth. Postpartum preeclampsia often occurs within 48 hours of childbirth and if left untreated can cause seizures, strokes and other serious complications (Mayo Clinic Staff, 2018).

There I was back in the hospital in Ohio, away from my newborn daughter, away from my mother and mother-in-law, bed bound and afraid. I was in the hospital for about four days. After my discharge, I still imagined that I would resume a blissful postpartum period. I would go home, nurse my newborn, bond with my baby, get back in shape, lose the baby weight, and be the perfect mom. That didn't happen, because once I got back home I still couldn't get the baby to latch on without it elevating my blood pressure and causing excruciating pain. My husband had to return to work. My mother and mother-in-law eventually had to return to Georgia and Maryland, respectively. I was home alone and lonely. I wasn't taking care of myself and may have bathed every other day. It was horrible! I had limited contact with people other than my husband. Instead of losing weight, I maintained the weight gained during pregnancy. Instead of feeling confident about motherhood, I felt unprepared and frightened.

My depression and anxiety during my second and third pregnancy and postpartum period was not as severe and didn't last as long. Right after the birth of my second child, I was completing my fellowship training and able to move back to the peach state of Georgia. "Georgia was on my mind!" and where most of my immediate family resided. It was great because I was closer to my parents, sisters, and brother! My support system magnified. In hindsight, this may have been one of the reasons my anxiety and depression wasn't as severe and didn't last as long. When my second oldest turned three years old, I started to get that itch! What itch, you may be asking. That 'I want another baby!' itch. So my husband and I tried and were successful getting pregnant with the third baby. I thought, 'Now our family is complete! We have our caboose!' Boy, was I wrong!

Now there are three! Not too big and not too small. However, I found out quickly that having two was not the same as having three children! You might be thinking, "*Duh*," but I believed the hype/myth that many other moms say, "Oh, having three children is about the same as having two!" Not in my case. I felt more overwhelmed and less on top of things. I felt my job was taking too much of my time from my family and from me! I was growing increasingly more resentful toward my job and contemplated leaving it many times. However, the "job security," "benefits," and, I admit, the unknown kept me there—despite feeling burnt out and unappreciated.

Spring of 2017, my husband and I were so excited when the youngest was about to graduate from pre-k! You know what that meant? NO MORE DAYCARE COST! Woo hoo! I was 40 years old by that time and thinking "Okay, I'm about to enter into another stage in my life!" I was becoming antsy, fed up, and burnt out at my job of eight years. I got tired of feeling unappreciated and tired of feeling like I was in a rat race. I spent so much time giving to others and not replenishing myself. I felt like I was failing as a wife and mother, often getting home and not having the energy to cook, clean, or help with homework. I felt like I was being a poor role model and doing a poor job as a mother. I found it difficult to invest time in building my business. I was no longer taking the time to nurture my interests, keep my hair done, decorate my house, which had always been a hobby, and the list goes on.

It was time for a change, so I built up enough courage and gave my job notice. My plan was to create my own schedule which would allow me to nurture and redis-cover my interests, spend more time with my daughters and husband, and nurture my private practice. I was riding high, proud of myself and relieved because I finally did it! I felt I was gaining momentum in reinvesting in myself, reclaiming and rediscovering me. I would have more time for myself, my business, my husband and my children. I was stepping into the arena of self-employment, which meant I would be responsible for the cost of my own health insurance, malpractice insurance, and there are no paid vacation days. Bottom line, if I don't work, I won't get paid. But let's go!

By the end of June 2017, I felt the momentum come to a halt. Well, it slowed down at least. My husband and I decided to do a staycation in Atlanta in celebration of our 16th wedding anniversary. This was the first time in a while we were doing something without the children (three children by now), but something wasn't right. I was experiencing changes in my body that was out of the ordinary, so I decided to take a pregnancy test. I went into the hotel restroom. My heart was pounding, and butterflies were dancing in my stomach. I was feeling anxious. I took the test and the stick immediately turned positive. I took another test. Same result. I burst into tears. Instead of being happy, I was sad, terrified, and feeling guilty. I remember thinking, "How am I going to take care of four kids when I'm barely hanging on and taking care of three? What's going to happen to all our family and business plans? Plus, I'm over 40!"

I walked out of the bathroom with tears pouring down my face. I probably had the ugly face cry. I said to my husband, "I'm pregnant! We can't afford another child! I'm struggling with the three we already have!" My husband didn't know how to react or what to say, so he kept silent. I immediately called my parents wailing and crying, then I called my close friend and daycare provider, wailing and crying! (I had to secure my spot because her daycare fills up quickly!) I'm sure I called a few more people (most likely my sisters). Everyone listened and tried to reassure me that everything was going to be okay, but I wasn't convinced. I was only thinking about the negative possibilities, which were driven by my anxiety and fear.

I was in shock for seven out of the nine months that I was pregnant. I had a difficult time accepting the fact that I was 40 years old and having another baby. As the ninth month approached, I became increasingly more anxious because I knew the postpartum period was coming. I knew the chances of experiencing postpartum depression were very high as I had experienced it after each of my previous children. I wanted it to be different this time around.

Like clockwork, around the fourth week post-delivery, my old uninvited guests, depression and anxiety, arrived. I worried about affording our utilities, the groceries, and daycare. The car was on its last leg, so how were we going to get around? Then, while still on unpaid maternity leave, my contract telemedicine job emailed me and said they found a provider to see their patients in person, so they no longer needed my services. It was like someone punched me in the gut. I was reminded of the cold and cruel world of business. It came at a very vulnerable time. The worse time!

So I was without an income and living off my savings. I was overcome with worry and instead of taking time to really recover, I started looking for other contract opportunities. I was becoming increasingly more depressed, irritable, and distant. My sister (also a physician) was just about to complete a coaching program and invited me to her graduation. The coaching experience transformed her life and she wanted me to experience a transformation too! I realized that whether I was ready or not, things had to change and transform. They say when one door closes, another door opens. I eventually ended up joining the coaching program. I guess the door wasn't wide open until the day my oldest daughter brought to my attention the change she observed in me. That was the moment I opened that new door WIDE OPEN.

From my experience, I realized that depression and anxiety during pregnancy is not discussed enough. Many women, including myself hide the truth, in fear of being considered unfit and "crazy" (Janice H. Goodman, 2009). It seemed as if the only time it is discussed is when there's a news headline of a mother who either hurt herself or hurt her children, even though those scenarios are the exception. I wore a figurative mask to hide the shame and embarrassment that I was depressed and anxious. I thought, "I'm a psychiatrist! I'm not supposed to feel depressed and anxious!" Somehow, I thought it reflected my competency. I began working on my mindset and realized that wearing this mask was perpetuating the depression and anxiety. Wearing the mask was hindering my growth. Once I removed my mask, I felt vulnerable, yet empowered and inspired. Thus, I desire to help women like me who have struggled with postpartum depression and anxiety feel empowered and inspired too. Empowered to speak their truth out loud and unapologetically—inspired to be proactive and seek the support and/or treatment needed so they can obtain mental health wellness individually and as a family.

I wrote this book to encourage mothers and their families to prepare for the postpartum period, aka "fourth trimester," in advance of delivery. Many women are ashamed, embarrassed, and feel that post-partum depression is a character flaw or weakness. Consequently, they suffer silently for extended periods of time. Additionally, I want to help increase the knowledge and understanding for mothers and their families about perinatal depression and anxiety, so we can decrease its stigma. Decreasing the stigma may help you and others seek the help needed. I want you to be informed and prepared to overcome postpartum depression and/or anxiety because your wellbeing and the wellbeing of your baby and family depends on it. Join me and remove the mask too!

PREHAB BEFORE POSTPARTUM: WHAT IS PREHAB?

Rehab vs. Prehab

Most people have heard of the term rehab. "Rehab" is short for rehabilitation. Rehabilitation is a treatment that is designed to help facilitate recovery from an illness, injury, or disease. It's used to help people achieve higher levels of function, independence, and quality of life. People often participate in rehabilitation after a surgery or injury to regain function or abilities. Others enter substance abuse rehabilitation to combat addictions, or psychiatric rehabilitation to promote recovery and improvement in the quality of life of individuals who have been diagnosed with a mental illness that has caused significant impairment in their lives (Psychiatric Rehabilitation, n.d.). But have you heard of prehab? My guess is no.

What is prehab? Prehab is the abbreviated term for prehabilitation, "a process that is designed to improve a person's physical and psychological health in <u>anticipation</u> of an upcoming stressor." It occurs after diagnosis but before treatment. It is a proactive approach, not a reactive approach (Malcolm A. West, 2017). The stressor could be an upcoming surgery or procedure. Or maybe there is no injury and you just want to engage in preventative exercises and strength training to prevent potential injuries.

Prehab is a term and concept that was born out of sports medicine, orthopedic medicine, and physical medicine rehabilitation. It usually occurs after an individual has been diagnosed with an ailment and before the treatment (or surgery). The goal of prehabilitation is to proactively improve the person's physical and/or mental state in preparation for a known or potential stressor. Prehabilitation has been shown to improve outcomes and reduce recovery time (Karen Pechman, 2014). Essentially, the more fit or prepared you are before the stressor (surgery, etc.), the quicker you will recover (Karen Pechman, 2014).

Early studies looking at prehab focused on just physical rehabilitation, such as physical exercise and endurance training. The approach to prehabilitation has since evolved to a more wholistic approach to include physical, nutrition, and psychological health. The physical approach may focus on strengthening, improving your core, balance, and endurance. The nutritional approach looks to determine what you need nutritionally to optimize your health because there are certain nutrients that may help with mental or physical wellbeing (Malcolm A. West, 2017). Finally, the psychological approach is important because your psychological wellbeing impacts your physical state and vice versa. Improving your psychological state may improve your ability to cope, which may reduce your stress level and positively impact your recovery.

Prehab for Postpartum

"Prehabilitation" is not usually used in disciplines other than the ones listed above. In my opinion it is a concept that could be used to improve the outcomes during pregnancy and after pregnancy. There has been a shift in the field of pregnancy. There are more discussions occurring to figure out ways to improve and optimize the health of women and infants. Historically, more attention has been placed on the antenatal period than the postpartum period. Antenatal period is the time before birth and during pregnancy (also known as prenatal). I had planned everything up until delivery, but nothing beyond that point. It is as if the postpartum period is an afterthought. We need to stop looking at it as if it's something separate, and look at the postpartum period as a continuation, which is why many now refer to it as the "fourth trimester." Many healthcare providers, like myself and health organizations, are working to redefine postpartum care.

The American College of Obstetricians and Gyne-cologist (ACOG) now have a list of recommendations to optimize postpartum care (May 2018). Some of their recommendations are as follows:

▶ "To optimize the health of women and infants, post-partum care should become an ongoing process, rather than a single encounter, with services and support tailored to each woman's individual needs."

▶ "All woman should ideally have contact with a ma-ternal care provider within the first three weeks post-partum. This initial assessment should be followed up with ongoing care as needed, concluding with a comprehensive postpartum visit no later than 12 weeks after birth."

▸ "The comprehensive postpartum visit should include a full assessment of physical, social, and psychological well-being."

▸ "Anticipatory guidance should begin during pregnancy with development of a postpartum care plan that addresses the transition to parenthood and well woman care."

The last recommendation, "anticipatory guidance should begin during pregnancy with development of a postpartum care plan…." (Optimizing Postpartum Care, 2018) is why I suggest prehab for postpartum. If we can anticipate what some of the challenges will be, or anticipate what your needs will be, we may be able to plan ahead of time and incorporate protective factors or protective measures that could prevent or reduce negative outcomes in the postpartum period.

Motherly Thoughts

_____

_____

_____

_____

_____

_____

_____

_____

_____

_____

_____

_____

_____

_____

_____

_____

_____

Motherly Thoughts

Motherly Thoughts

Motherly Thoughts

_____

_____

_____

_____

_____

_____

_____

_____

_____

_____

_____

_____

_____

_____

_____

_____

Motherly Thoughts

WHAT IS PERINATAL DEPRESSION?

Pregnancy for many is a very joyous time, but it is not joyous for everyone. Not all pregnancies are the idealized picture of perfection often portrayed on television. When I was pregnant, I imagined what pregnancy and the postpartum period would be like, imagining I would be the perfect mother and perfect wife. In my mind, I would have an uncomplicated birth experience, breastfeed without issues, and be Betty Crocker of sorts. None of that was what I experienced. Labor was challenging. A few days after delivery I ended up in the ICU after developing preeclampsia and I was unsuccessful at breastfeeding my first born. I was devastated about the turn of events and ended up developing postpartum depression and postpartum anxiety. I could have benefitted from a prehab postpartum plan. But before discussing what goes into prehabbing for postpartum, let's first discuss what we are trying to prevent!

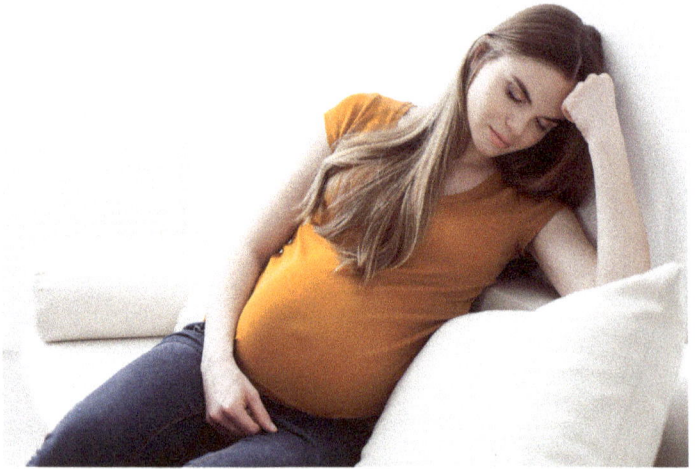

Depression that occurs during or within a year following pregnancy is frequently referred to as perinatal depression. Perinatal refers to the time prior to delivery and after delivery of the baby. Perinatal depression is one of many perinatal mental health illnesses women may suffer from. Perinatal mental illnesses are a group of disorders/illnesses that may have started before, during, and after pregnancy.

The mental health of a pregnant and postpartum woman is very important because it impacts your emotional, psychological, and social well-being. It influences how you think, feel, and act. It also affects how we deal with stress, relate to others, and what we choose to do or not do. I recall after my first child, feeling depressed, isolated, and anxious. I also felt inadequate and like I failed my daughter. Those feelings, in turn, impacted and delayed my bonding experience with her. Fortunately, because of my knowledge and profession, I was aware of the signs and symptoms. I knew the difference between postpartum blues and postpartum depression. However, thousands of other women and their families don't know what to look for. Many don't know how to treat the symptoms or are ashamed of what they are experiencing. As a result, many suffer silently and alone. Untreated perinatal mental health issues can negatively impact the health of the family, mother, and infant. Thus, it's extremely important to identify psychiatric illnesses during this time.

Types of perinatal depression include: antenatal depression and postpartum depression. Antenatal depression and postpartum depression will usually look like regular depression (Pearson, 2018). Depression is a mood disorder that causes a persistent feeling of sadness and loss of interest in things you use to enjoy doing. It affects how you feel, think, and behave. It can cause other emotional and physical symptoms. Depression will last at least two weeks and will be associated with some or all the symptoms listed below most of the day, nearly every day:

▶ Sadness, feelings of hopelessness, feeling empty inside, feeling worthless or excessive guilt

▶ Crying episodes, constantly feeling tired, everything seems to take a lot of effort and energy

▶ Irritability or frustrations over little things, anger outbursts

▶ Sleep disturbance: sleeping too much or not sleeping enough

▶ Appetite disturbance: reduced appetite that may be accompanied by weight loss or increased appetite or craving that is associated with weight gain

▶ Poor concentration, slowed thinking, slow body movements and speech

▶ Ruminating: constantly thinking about the past (i.e. failures)

▶ Loss of pleasure in most things such as people, hobbies, sex, or sports

▶ Frequent or recurrent thoughts of death, suicidal thoughts, suicide attempts

Depression is the most common mood disorder, and it is about twice as common in women compared to men. It is especially common among women during child bearing ages. Depression can be mild, moderate, or severe and can be very debilitating for many women. Approximately 14%- 23% of pregnant women and 5% to 25% of postpartum women experience depression are not aware of the signs and symptoms. Less than half of the women diagnosed with postpartum depression will get treated. Postpartum depression persists for over seven months after delivery for 25%–50% of women, and many remain depressed after one year. Perinatal depression is prevalent, under-recognized, and undertreated.

When you're depressed, it will negatively impact your level of functioning. For instance, when I was depressed I had no desire to do anything other than lay around. I recall maybe taking a bath every other day, I lost interest in writing, and there was a change in my appetite. Sometimes depression can become so severe, some women may experience psychotic symptoms. Psychotic symptoms may include: feeling paranoid, delusional, and experiencing hallucinations (seeing or hearing things that aren't there).

Postpartum Blues vs. Postpartum Depression

So what's the difference between postpartum depression and postpartum blues? Well, postpartum blues is considered a normal occurrence. In fact, approximately 50% to 80% of new mothers will experience it. Signs may include depressed mood, anxiety, tearfulness, irritability, poor appetite and sleep problems. These symptoms are usually mild and will resolve on their own within 10 to 14 days. One in four women who experience postpartum blues will go on to develop postpartum depression. Many women lose track of time. They notice a few of the symptoms and chalk it up to postpartum blues, but actually have postpartum depression.

If you experience postpartum depression, it is important to distinguish it from bipolar disorder. Bipolar is also a mood disorder. A person with bipolar can have depressive episodes, mania, hypomania, and mixed episodes.

A person with postpartum bipolar can initially present as depressed then develop mania and/or psychosis. It's important to distinguish between the two, because the treatment is different, and the depression medication treatment could potentially trigger or exacerbate bipolar disorder.

Evaluation

If your doctor suspects perinatal depression, they will most likely have you complete The Edinburgh Postnatal Depression Scale (EPDS). The EPDS is the most commonly used self-report instrument for the assessment of postpartum depression. It is not used to diagnosis but to identify those at risk. The EPDS will usually be administered by your obstetrician, but it can also be administered by your child's pediatrician as well. It is the mental health professional who will perform a detailed evaluation and diagnosis.

Motherly Thoughts

Motherly Thoughts

Motherly Thoughts

_____

_____

_____

_____

_____

_____

_____

_____

_____

_____

_____

_____

_____

_____

_____

_____

_____

_____

Motherly Thoughts

Motherly Thoughts

WHAT CAUSES POSTPARTUM DEPRESSION?

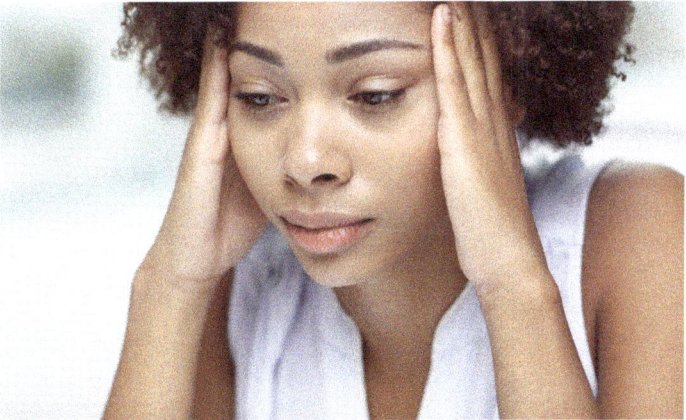

The cause of postpartum depression is unknown. There are several possible causes, but it may vary from person to person. One of the possible causes is referred to as the hormonal theory. During pregnancy, levels of the female hormones estrogen and progesterone gradually increase to the highest they'll ever be. Yet, in the first 24 hours after childbirth, hormone levels quickly drop back to the level before pregnancy. Estrogen and progesterone impacts parts of the brain that deal with emotions. It's thought that their rapid decrease may trigger symptoms of postpartum depression.

Many believe that it is the interplay between biological, psychological, and social factors that lead to the development of postpartum depression. Biological factors are things within your body's makeup that impact the way you and your body behaves. Examples of biological factors are hormones and genes (what you have inherited from your family). It could also be possible that your brain doesn't produce enough serotonin (chemical involved with the development of depression). Psychological factors are your thoughts, feelings, personality, and attitude. Examples of a psychological factors are coping strategies (poor adjustment to motherhood), and the way you think. Social factors are things that affect the way you live, like the loss of a job, pregnancy, relationship problems, lack of a support system, family structure, or religion. When these types of things occur together, there is an additive effect that increases the chance of developing postpartum depression. Look at the balance scale below. The more things that put you at risk, the higher your chances are to develop postpartum depression.

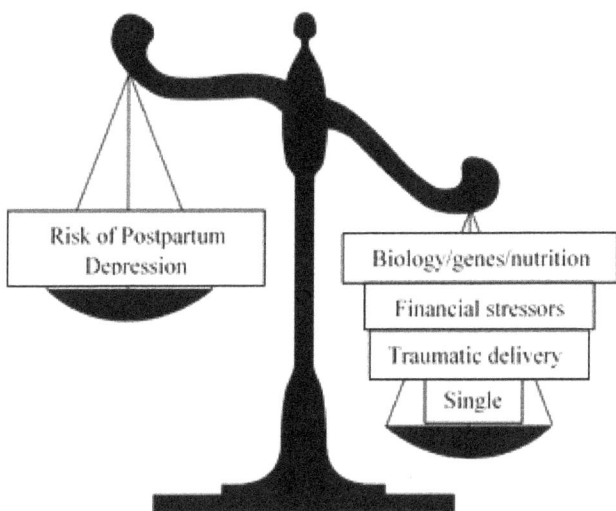

Risk of Postpartum Depression

Biology/genes/nutrition

Financial stressors

Traumatic delivery

Single

Management

The treatment can begin before the postpartum period. Interventions that target women at risk has helped prevent postpartum in some women. Some of you have chronic depression or have developed antenatal depression. Being proactive and starting treatment during the antenatal period may help improve postpartum outcomes.

Treatment is usually talk therapy, medication, and/ or electroconvulsive therapy. They can be used alone or together.

Talk Therapy

Interpersonal psychotherapy (IPT) when started during pregnancy has been found to help reduce depression during the postpartum period. There was a study conducted where depressed pregnant moms were provided massage therapy or twice weekly yoga over a 12-week period, and it significantly improved their depression.

Management and treatment for postpartum depression depends on the severity of the symptoms, the type of depression, and whether or not the mother is breastfeeding.

If you have been diagnosed with mild to moderate depression, the treatment of choice is psychotherapy. Two types of therapy have helped reduce postpartum depression symptoms: cognitive behavioral therapy and interpersonal therapy. These therapies will usually occur over a 10- to 20-week period.

Medication

If you have been diagnosed with moderate to severe depression, antidepressant medication, with or without therapy, is recommended during pregnancy or during the postpartum period if needed. Even if you strongly prefer not to use medication in the perinatal period, the risk to the baby when depression goes untreated suggests that lack of treatment may be more detrimental to the infant.

If you are planning on breastfeeding, it's imperative that you and your provider select a medication that will have minimal effect on the infant. All antidepressants pass from the mother to breast milk, but some will be less concentrated then others. For example, Sertraline is thought to be relatively safe because it has less passage into the milk and fewer reported side effects on the baby. It's best to try to use the least amount of medicine possible. Babies and mothers who are taking an antidepressant need to be followed closely. It may also be helpful to consult a lactation consultant and pediatrician if you're planning on breastfeeding. Treatment can be provided by your primary care physician or a psychiatrist. If you are suicidal or homicidal, then hospitalization may be needed.

Electroconvulsive therapy

Electroconvulsive therapy (ECT) is a type of treatment used for severe depression. It is specifically for people who are experiencing thoughts of self-harm and severe symptoms that are not responding to medication. "Electroconvulsive therapy (ECT) is a procedure done under general anesthesia in which small electric currents are passed through the brain, intentionally triggering a brief seizure. ECT seems to cause changes in brain chemistry that can quickly reverse symptoms of certain mental illnesses." Electroconvulsive therapy is still being used—more in Europe than the United States—and it may be the most effective short-term treatment for some patients with depressive symptoms, a newly published review in *The Lancet* suggests.

Motherly Thoughts

_____

_____

_____

_____

_____

_____

_____

_____

_____

_____

_____

_____

_____

_____

_____

_____

_____

_____

Motherly Thoughts

Motherly Thoughts

Motherly Thoughts

WHAT IS PERINATAL ANXIETY?

Perinatal anxiety is experienced during or after pregnancy. While most people have heard about postpartum depression, many are not aware of and do not talk about perinatal anxiety. Perinatal anxiety is often not diagnosed because the anxiety is attributed as being a normal reaction to pregnancy and birth. Also, many women don't speak up because of the stigma associated with being diagnosed with a mental illness.

Perinatal anxiety is actually more common than perinatal depression. In fact, prenatal anxiety has been identified as a strong predictor of postpartum depression. Just like depression during pregnancy, anxiety during pregnancy is associated with adverse pregnancy outcomes such as miscarriage, preeclampsia, preterm delivery, and low birth weight. Furthermore, children of highly anxious mothers have twice the risk for developing ADHD.

There are several different types of anxiety disorders frequently seen during or after pregnancy. They are listed below:

Type of anxiety disorder	Symptoms
Generalized anxiety disorder	Excessive worrying about everything from A to Z. Occurring most days and you have difficulty controlling the worry. I often describe them as the "worry warts!" Headaches, backaches, and irritability can be also be seen.
Obsessive Compulsive Disorder	Unwanted thoughts or fears, thoughts or fears that keep popping in your mind and causes anxiety and/or makes you feel like you must carry out certain routines or rituals to feel less anxious.
Panic disorder	Frequent distinct periods of intense anxiety or fear; it feels like you're out of control.

Post-traumatic Stress Disorder	Intense anxiety that occurs following a traumatic event witnessed or personally experienced where you feel like your reliving the trauma (nightmares, flashbacks, hallucinations). You try to avoid people, places, thoughts, or situations that remind you of the trauma; easily aroused (jumpy, quick to anger, rapid pulse, etc.) and experiencing a lot of negative thoughts and feelings.
Social phobia	An extreme fear of being criticized by others or fear of being humiliated. Thus, you might try to avoid public situations or social situations (avoid speaking to people or eating in public)
Specific phobia	Intense fear of a specific thing or situation (i.e. fear of needles, fear of bugs, fear of heights)
Tokophobia	fear of childbirth

Common Signs and Symptoms

Common signs and symptoms among most anxiety disorders include:

▶ worry or fear that leads moms to check on her baby constantly

▶ worry or fear that may prevent moms from going out in public with their baby

▶ worry and fearful thoughts that intrude and get in the way of completing daily tasks or routines

▶ constant fear and worry

▶ feeling irritable, restless, or on edge

▶ heart palpitations, chest tightness, tense and tight muscles

▶ unable to relax

▶ taking long times to fall asleep

What Causes Perinatal Anxiety?

Just like perinatal depression, there is no single cause of perinatal anxiety. It's most likely due to a combination of biological, psychological, and social factors. Remember biological factors are things within your body's makeup that impact the way you and your body behaves. Psychological factors are your thoughts, feelings, personality, and attitude. Social factors are things that affect the way you live like the loss of a job, relationship problems, lack of a support system, family structure, or religion. The more biological, psychological, and social factors that occur at once will increase risk of developing perinatal anxiety.

Evaluation

Perinatal anxiety can occur during or after pregnancy at any time. Moms in the perinatal period should be screened on a regular basis (more than once). The Edinburgh Postnatal Depression Scale is usually used to not only identify possible depression in the perinatal period, it is also used to identify perinatal anxiety as well. However, it is not used to diagnose perinatal anxiety but to identify those who are at risk of developing perinatal anxiety and depression. It should only be used with a qualified mental health provider who can then assess and provide a diagnosis.

Management

Some of the treatment for perinatal anxieties may be similar to perinatal depression. Usually the treatment for anxiety will fall under two categories: talk therapy and medication.

Talk therapy is often beneficial for mild to moderate anxiety. The therapy will target the mother's thoughts feelings and behaviors. It will also strive to help improve the mom's coping strategies. If the anxiety symptoms are severe, talk therapy and medication are usually recommended. The safety of the medication for the fetus and/or infant (if breastfeeding) need to be taken into consideration.

Motherly Thoughts

_____

_____

_____

_____

_____

_____

_____

_____

_____

_____

_____

_____

_____

_____

_____

_____

_____

_____

Motherly Thoughts

Motherly Thoughts

_____

_____

_____

_____

_____

_____

_____

_____

_____

_____

_____

_____

_____

_____

_____

_____

_____

_____

_____

Motherly Thoughts

WHAT ARE THE RISK FACTORS?

Some of you may be wondering, "What is a risk factor?" A risk factor is something that increases your chances of developing a disease and getting injured (World Health Organization, 2018). Now you may be wondering, "Am I at risk?" Well, some of you are more at risk than others. The more risk factors that you identify, the higher your chances of developing postpartum depression or anxiety.

In hindsight, I realized that I had a number of the risk factors for developing depression and anxiety during and after pregnancy. As mentioned, I'm a mother of four beautiful girls. I experienced postpartum depression and anxiety with my first daughter and antenatal and postpartum depression and anxiety with my last daughter.

Shortly after delivering my first daughter, I was diagnosed with pre-eclampsia and was hospitalized in the ICU (Intensive Care Unit). This was just days after bringing her home from the hospital. Remember, within 24 hours we have a drastic reduction in our hormone levels, and within the first two weeks most women will experience "baby blues." That alone sets the tone, because I was admitted to the hospital during a very vulnerable time. Going to the ICU disrupted the initial bonding time, and once I returned home, I was unable to breastfeed because of the excruciating pain which would elevate my blood pressure. Additionally, I didn't live near any family (minimal social support), I was experiencing some anxiety in anticipation of meeting my daughter and I was in medical residency training at the time which can be very stressful.

My last pregnancy was a "surprise baby." It occurred during a time of *great* transition. Prior to finding out I was pregnant, I was experiencing physician burn-out at my then current job, and I submitted my resignation to my job of eight years, deciding to focus on my private practice and work independently. I knew I would lose some of the benefits of working for someone else, but I was looking forward to having more time for me and having more time for my family. I recall feeling depressed and anxious during the pregnancy. This was not the optimal time to be having another baby, I thought. I was in shock for the first seven months! I often would say to myself, "I can't believe I'm starting all over again!" "Is this really happening?" "I'm struggling to keep up with 3 children… now I'll have 4 children!"

So, the risk factors that I identified for my first pregnancy were maternal anxiety, life stress, and lack of social support. The risk factors I identified for the last pregnancy were unexpected/unplanned pregnancy, depression during pregnancy, anxiety during pregnancy, stress during pregnancy, history of high blood pressure post-delivery, previous history of postpartum depression, and breastfeeding difficulties. Take a look below and identify your risk factors.

Risk Factors for Depression and Anxiety During Pregnancy

▶ Maternal anxiety

▶ Life stress (relationship conflicts, employment issues, etc.)

▶ History of depression

▶ Lack of social support

▶ Unintended pregnancy

- Medicaid insurance

- Lower income/ financial issues

- Lower education

- Smoking

- Single Status

- Poor relationship quality

- Family history

- Health issues

- Multiple children

Risk Factors for Postpartum Depression and Anxiety

- Depression during pregnancy

- Anxiety during pregnancy

- Experiencing stressful life events during pregnancy or the early postpartum period (Did you struggle with getting pregnant? Baby born with special needs, Are you in a toxic relationship?)

▸ Traumatic birth experience (for example, complications during delivery)

▸ Preterm birth/infant admission to neonatal intensive care

▸ Lower levels of social support (family, friends, etc.)

▸ Single Status

▸ Previous history of depression

▸ Breastfeeding problems

▸ Family history anxiety or depression

▸ Family history of perinatal anxiety or depression

▸ Previous mood reaction to hormonal changes—i.e., PMS, etc.

▸ Previous pregnancy or infant loss

▸ Becoming pregnant during teen years

▸ History of thyroid imbalance or diabetes

▸ Crisis in job, finances, or housing

Motherly Thoughts

_____

_____

_____

_____

_____

_____

_____

_____

_____

_____

_____

_____

_____

_____

_____

_____

_____

_____

_____

Motherly Thoughts

_____

_____

_____

_____

_____

_____

_____

_____

_____

_____

_____

_____

_____

_____

_____

_____

Motherly Thoughts

Motherly Thoughts

_____

_____

_____

_____

_____

_____

_____

_____

_____

_____

_____

_____

_____

_____

_____

_____

_____

_____

_____

Motherly Thoughts

OUTCOMES OF POSTPARTUM DEPRESSION AND POSTPARTUM ANXIETY

For those who are reluctant to seek help or are convinced that their symptoms are just mild, and they'll go away on their own, I'd like to share what could happen if you don't. The most eye-opening thing for me occurred when I began to see the change in my oldest daughter's mood and behavior. She appeared more irritable than the normal preteen, especially towards her sisters. She appeared more guarded and less open and playful. In hindsight, perhaps she was just mirroring what she observed in me! One day she asked, "Mommy, when are you going to go back to your normal self?" She went on to share that she had noticed a difference in me and that I seemed angry all the time. It stopped me in my tracks. Her candidness helped me to stop and reflect. I had not realized how my struggles with my own issues of trying to navigate my new responsibilities might be affecting her or the rest of the family. That was a wakeup call.

There are long term and short-term consequences of untreated perinatal depression and anxiety. Untreated perinatal depression and anxiety can lead to several negative outcomes. It doesn't just impact the mother. It impacts the newborn, your partner, your other children...anyone you potentially meet or interact with. As discussed before, depression can be debilitating and change the way you feel, think, and act. It can cause you to not be as in tune with your loved ones or cause you to be less patient and more irritable. It may also impact your ability to concentrate, therefore making it more difficult to retain information. Depression and anxiety can also cause you to be more distracted, isolative, and feel unconfident. I recall feeling inadequate as a mother. I would lose my temper with my older children and feel guilt shortly afterwards. I found myself in a never-ending cycle of sadness, irritability, and guilt. Studies have shown that antenatal depression during the second trimester and postpartum depression may cause changes in the child's brain structure and increase their risk of developing depression and anxiety later (Peckel, 2016). This suggests that the second trimester and postpartum are vulnerable times in the development of the baby's brain. Infants may appear less social and could suffer developmental delays (for example social and language delays). Some of the long-term impacts on the infant and other children also included: ADHD (Attention Deficit Hyperactivity Disorder), learning disorders, lower IQ, difficulty regulating their behavior, and anxiety disorders (Canadian Paediatric Society, 2004).

Depending on how severe the postpartum depression or anxiety is, it can lead to a neglected home environment for the infant and any other children in the home. Postpartum depression and anxiety may interfere with mother-infant interaction, and it can make it more difficult for the mom to interpret cues from the baby (Pat F. Bass III, 2018). Since the baby can't talk, parents rely on behavioral and vocal cues to understand the baby's desires and needs. If the mother is depressed or anxious, she may be less attentive, and this could interrupt or jeopardize secure and healthy attachment (Nur, 2018).

In the chart listed below are possible negative outcomes that could arise because of untreated perinatal depression and anxiety.

Risk of untreated Antenatal Mental illness	Risk of untreated Postpartum Mental Illness
Less active in prenatal treatment	
Risky behaviors such as smoking or substance abuse	
Infants admitted to neonatal intensive care	
Risk of preterm birth and low birth rate	
Risk of pre-eclampsia	
	Weight retention
Diabetes	

▶ Absence of breastfeeding may trigger postpartum mood disorder

▶ Perinatal depression and anxiety may lead to decrease initiation of breastfeeding as well as decrease duration of breastfeeding.

▶ Early difficulty with breastfeeding may lead to postpartum depression and anxiety

▶ Maternal suicide

▶ Infanticide

▶ Decreased maternal sensitivity

- ▶ Attachment and bonding with infant.

- ▶ Marital problems

- ▶ Relationship with others

- ▶ Decrease functioning which can impact job performance.

- ▶ Could influence depression in fathers-Paternal postpartum depression.

- ▶ Untreated antenatal depression and anxiety

- ▶ Untreated depression or anxiety during the antenatal and postpartum period increases the risk of long term mood and anxiety disorders down the line.

If you deal with antenatal (during pregnancy) depression, you are less likely to participate in the recommended prenatal care practices. You are also at increased risk of engaging in unhealthy ways of coping and risky behaviors such as substance abuse and smoking. As a result, it puts you at risk of having complications during your pregnancy and after pregnancy, such as pre-term labor or low birth weight. Additionally, not treating depression during pregnancy will increase your chance of having postpartum depression. This is important because postpartum depression is one of the greatest causes of death among women. Postpartum depression increases the risk of maternal suicide and infanticide (murder of infant). If you don't treat depression or anxiety during pregnancy or postpartum (fourth trimester), you will increase your risk of developing long-term mood disorders down the line.

Paternal Postpartum Depression (PPD)

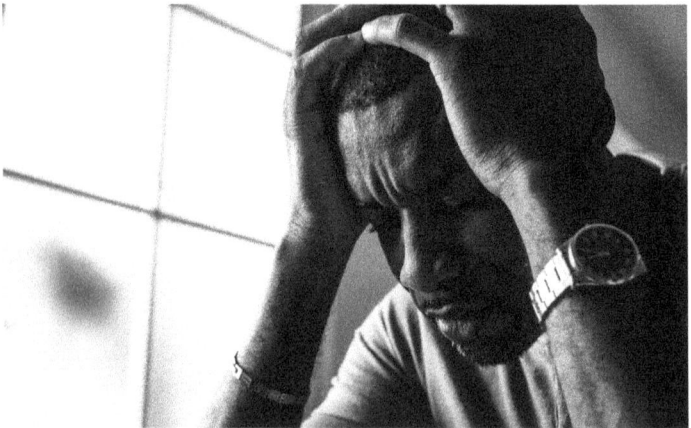

Before we move on, I want to briefly discuss paternal postpartum depression. Yes! Your eyes are not deceiving you. Paternal postpartum depression (PPD) exists.

Postpartum depression has historically been considered an issue unique to the mother. However, fathers also experience it. They are not immune to the changes that occur after a child is born. They also must adjust to a new norm. One out of every ten men will get depressed shortly before or after the birth of their newborn, and younger dads are at a higher risk. Approximately 5% of first-time fathers become depressed during pregnancy, 5% were depressed three months postpartum, and approximately 24% of fathers were depressed a year after childbirth. Common symptoms seen in paternal postpartum depression is depressed or low mood, irritability, and feelings of helplessness. It can co-occur with anxiety and OCD (obsessive compulsive disorder). Paternal postpartum depression is believed to develop more gradually over time than postpartum depression in mothers.

Multiple paternal postpartum depression risk factors have been divided into biological and social (or ecological) categories. Regarding biological risk factors, there is some research that suggest changes in hormones as being possible risk factors. Not only do mothers go through hormonal changes during and after pregnancy, so do the fathers. Thus, some of those hormones may be associated with changes in mood, ability to bond with infant, and vulnerability (PILYOUNG KIM, 2007).

Other risk factors include: lack of support, feeling excluded from the bond observed between the mother and infant, and the most important risk factor is maternal antenatal and postnatal depression. Some fathers feel isolated and not a part of the bonding experience and can become jealous. Fathers may also become jealous of the mothers' bond with the infant (especially if breast-feeding is involved) and/or become jealous of the baby because the baby occupies and dominates the mother's attention. Often the mother and father can become depressed in the postpartum period at the same time. If both parents happen to be depressed at the same time, this would interfere with the normal development of the infant and other children in the home.

PPD has a negative impact on the family and can increase emotional and behavioral problems among their children and cause or exacerbate marital problems. Children of fathers dealing with postpartum depression have more behavioral problems and hyperactivity. This may affect boys more than girls. Paternal postpartum depression may disrupt children's development of a secure attachment with the father and cause more marital discord. Studies have shown that both mothers and fathers have reported feeling less satisfied in their marriage. Frequently, there's less intimacy and mothers may lose interest in sex. Additionally, some studies have also shown violence occurring for the first time between partners during the postpartum period.

Motherly Thoughts

_____

_____

_____

_____

_____

_____

_____

_____

_____

_____

_____

_____

_____

_____

_____

_____

_____

Motherly Thoughts

_____

_____

_____

_____

_____

_____

_____

_____

_____

_____

_____

_____

_____

_____

_____

_____

_____

Motherly Thoughts

Motherly Thoughts

_____

_____

_____

_____

_____

_____

_____

_____

_____

_____

_____

_____

_____

_____

_____

_____

_____

_____

_____

_____

Motherly Thoughts

PREHAB BEFORE POSTPARTUM (4TH TRIMESTER)

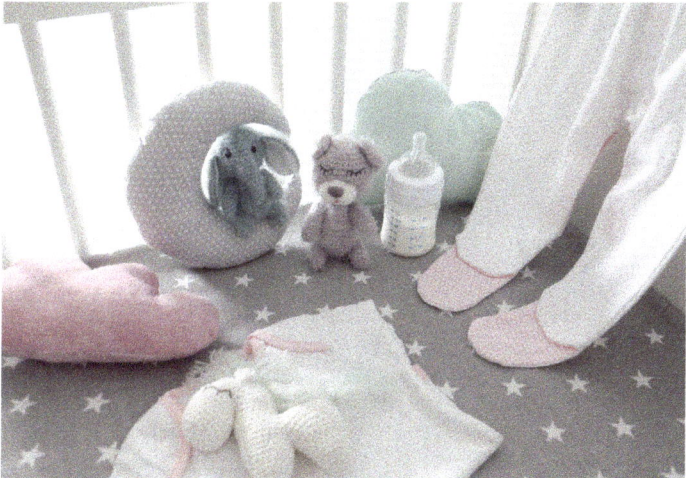

Pregnant women spend a lot of time preparing for the delivery. "What kind of music will I play, will it be a natural birth? Will I get an epidural, or will I have to have a

C-section? Who will be in the room with me?" We even pack our bags for our hospital stay in advance. We don't spend enough time planning for the postpartum period. For the working mother, we'll think about when we must return to work, or think about daycare plans, and not giving much thought or attention to the time immediately after delivery and the time leading back to work.

Historically, most of the preparation is geared toward the baby and not for you and most is in preparation for the birth and not the "fourth trimester" aka postpartum. We must find the balance and shift our mindset. The birth is not the finale. It's a chapter in the book of life, much like the wedding is not the marriage; it's just the precursor. To look at postpartum as if it's something unrelated and insignificant is a mistake. Additionally, we must recognize taking care of ourselves will allow us to be more prepared and able to care for our baby and family. As discussed in the previous chapter, there are short-term and long-term consequences of not recognizing, diagnosing, and treating perinatal mental health illnesses.

Increasingly more health organizations are encouraging women and health providers to plan for postpartum care. Many refer to this as the postpartum care plan, but I like to call it "Prehab for Postpartum!" Remember, prehab is known as "a process that was designed to improve a person's physical and psychological health in anticipation of an upcoming stressor." So those who have had children before know postpartum, even on a good day, can be challenging. What if there are some things we could anticipate and, in turn, plan for? Now I don't want to mislead you into thinking that prehabbing for postpartum will guarantee that you'll have a perfect postpartum period, or that you won't suffer from a perinatal mental health issue. What I'm proposing is that if we prepare ,we could lessen the stress. If we prepare, we might be able to reduce the severity of postpartum depression and/or anxiety, and for some prevent it. The goal is to plan so you won't forget about caring for you!

I still remember what my mom told me when I returned from the ICU and was desperate to master breastfeeding. My blood pressure was still coming down and every time I attempted to breast feed, my blood pressure would go back up, "If you don't take care of yourself," she said, "how are you going to take care of the baby?" Chronic high blood pressure can be fatal. Ladies, it's not the end of the world if you can't breastfeed your baby. You can still feed, love, nurture and care for your baby if he/she is bottle fed.

Remember, we all may have risk factors some of them are modifiable and others are not. If they are modifiable, that means they can be altered or changed. You can change or alter your support system; you can have an impact on your schedule. If they are non-modifiable, they are not able to be changed or altered. For instance, the things you cannot change would be your genes. You cannot change the fact that you inherited certain genes from each of your parents, and you can't change your height.

Let's prehab for postpartum by identifying the things that we can change and the things that could potentially lessen the stress of this very important moment in your life.

Motherly Thoughts

_____

_____

_____

_____

_____

_____

_____

_____

_____

_____

_____

_____

_____

_____

_____

_____

Motherly Thoughts

_____

_____

_____

_____

_____

_____

_____

_____

_____

_____

_____

_____

_____

_____

_____

_____

_____

Motherly Thoughts

Motherly Thoughts

GETTING STARTED ON YOUR PREHAB POSTPARTUM PLAN

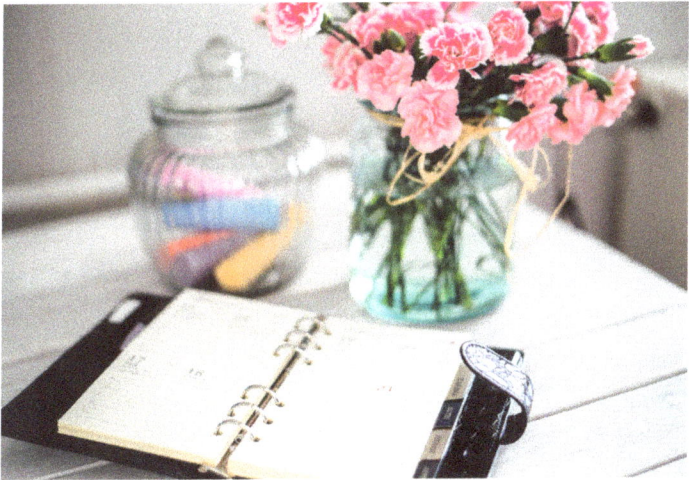

Your prehab is going to be uniquely yours. I have three recommendations in preparation for your prehab post-partum plan:

Step 1

Start as early as possible. If you are in a relationship, plan together because as we discussed earlier, your partner can develop postpartum depression and anxiety as well. Moms, you are not the only ones at risk. Remember, one out of every ten men will get depressed shortly before or after the birth of their newborn (Pat F. Bass III, 2018). Younger dads are at an even higher risk. So when recruiting the help of your partner, make sure the both of you take the time for self-care.

Having a support system is helpful. The earlier, the better. To avoid stressing at the last minute, I recommend that you use a calendar and a notebook. The calendar or notebook can be hardback or electronic.

Step 2

Identify what you want. There's nothing wrong with considering what you want. Remember one of the goals is to help you prioritize yourself, something you probably aren't use to doing. Maybe you want to get a massage at some point, or maybe get your hair and nails done. Perhaps you want some time to yourself to meditate or resume coaching or therapy. What would help lift your spirits? Think outside of the box!

Step 3

Identify what you (and your partner) need. There are things that you will need. For instance, you will need to identify a pediatrician. You will need to decide about vaccinations, feeding options, you will need to eat, you will need to bathe. You will need to have follow up appointments.

Your prehab plan may include your physical, psychosocial, and nutritional needs. There are a few things I want you to consider:

▶ Think about the things you will need, especially the first few weeks. One thing for sure, you will need REST! You will need to become creative. Find ways to get rest. Lack of sleep and rest can increase stress levels and put some people at risk of triggering manic episodes. Create a list of people (contact information) who might be able to assist you in the first couple of weeks. Maybe it's a postpartum doula or maybe a family member or friend. Is there someone who can come during the day or evening while you rest? They might be able to tend to other things, i.e. other children, cleaning, etc. while you rest. If you have other children, it's important to have support. You need to know where they will go when you go into labor. Is there anyone who can help them maintain their daily routine? I'm a mother of four now and each child has a different personality and each child has different needs. I had to figure out who was going to pick up the siblings from school and daycare? Who would take them to tutoring? Who was going to provide the housekeeping and complete the chores?

▶ You and your family (partner or children) will need to eat. You will need nutritious meals. You will likely be the main caregiver for the newborn. As a result, you won't have time to cook. What will you do? You can plan menus and go to the store before delivering and cook several meals and freeze them. Or you could identify meals that would be easy to prepare, like a crockpot dish. You could order groceries online and have them shipped to your home or identify affordable and healthy take-out options in advance. Perhaps you have friends and family who wouldn't mine preparing and delivering food to your home. There are a few web-based/online programs that will allow people to sign up and volunteer their time or volunteer to prepare a meal. If you start early, you can have people volunteer ahead of time and get reminders as their chosen date approaches. Maybe include the postpartum plan at the time of your baby shower (if you're having one) as an activity.

▶ Know in advance what your feeding options are for the baby. Will you breastfeed? Will you use formula? Which formula? If you are going to breastfeed, go ahead and list lactation consultant resources or maybe you have friends or family who are experts in breastfeeding.

▶ Finally, you have to think about things that will be specifically for feeding your spirit, your mental wellness and physical wellness. Who do you trust to watch the baby, so you can get rejuvenated? Maybe you want to go to the spa, or get your nails and hair done, or spend time with your partner. If you are at risk of developing postpartum depression and/or anxiety, it's important to identify your support system. Who are the people you can talk to? Who are the mental health professionals that you will likely see. Go ahead and make your appointment in advance, especially if you had antenatal depression or if you have a history of perinatal mental illnesses from previous pregnancies or suffered from depression/anxiety, etc. prior to pregnancy. Plan for your physical wellness ahead of time. Once you get the green light from your OB/GYN, you will already have an exercise plan in place. Consider hiring a personal trainer or purchasing a gym membership.

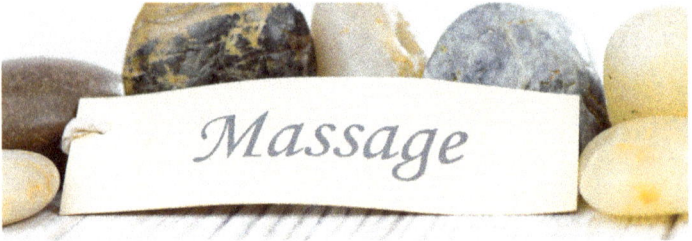

When creating your prehab postpartum plan, make sure you are specific about what your needs are and simultaneously be flexible. Be flexible, because despite planning there could be hiccups along the way. The advantage is that you've already thought about possible solutions way in advance, which gives you options.

Motherly Thoughts

_____

_____

_____

_____

_____

_____

_____

_____

_____

_____

_____

_____

_____

_____

_____

_____

_____

_____

Motherly Thoughts

_____

_____

_____

_____

_____

_____

_____

_____

_____

_____

_____

_____

_____

_____

_____

_____

_____

_____

Motherly Thoughts

_____

_____

_____

_____

_____

_____

_____

_____

_____

_____

_____

_____

_____

_____

_____

_____

_____

_____

Motherly Thoughts

CONCLUSION

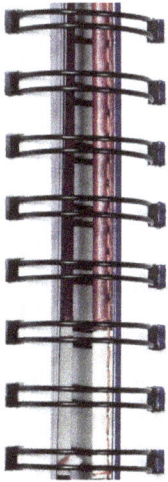

MY PLAN

So far, we discussed perinatal depression and anxiety: the signs, causes, how to detect it and treatment. We have discussed the consequences of not seeking treatment and identified risk factors. This will help you assess whether you or your family member is at risk of developing perinatal depression and anxiety. Then we discussed the importance of creating a prehab plan. Now it's time to implement it!

As discussed in the previous chapter, it would be helpful if you include your partner when developing a plan. If you don't have a partner, then identify someone such as a sibling, parent, friend or a doula who can help you. They will be helpful, not only in the development of the plan, but they will be essential in implementing the plan.

I have met so many women who just suffer through perinatal depression and two to five years down the line, they still are suffering because they ignored the signs because of being uninformed or embarrassed. They were embarrassed to express out loud that sometimes, "I feel like my child is a burden to me!" Embarrassment and shame often prevent women from seeking the help they need. This needs to change.

The consequences of not treating perinatal mental illnesses is great. It can negatively impact the physical health, mental health, and the safety of the mother and her family. Therefore, early screening and intervention is key. An integrated intervention that include the mental, physical, and social supports will be essential.

Some of you have experienced depression and/or anxiety and know firsthand how impairing depression and/or anxiety can be. Often you lose motivation and energy to carry out tasks. Well, perinatal depression or anxiety is not any different. You may need someone who will cheer you on and assist you if you don't have the energy or motivation to do it yourself.

Now that you have your plan and your team…get into action! Shed your mask. Congratulate yourself, because you're one step closer to a happier postpartum!

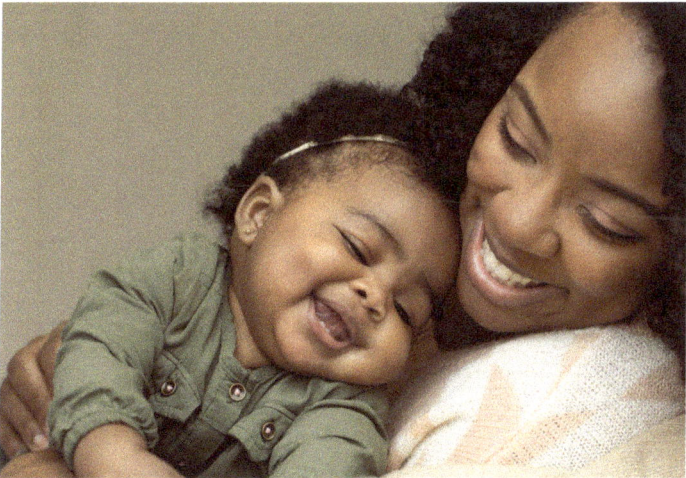

Motherly Thoughts

Motherly Thoughts

_____

_____

_____

_____

_____

_____

_____

_____

_____

_____

_____

_____

_____

_____

_____

_____

Motherly Thoughts

Motherly Thoughts

Motherly Thoughts

_____

_____

_____

_____

_____

_____

_____

_____

_____

_____

_____

_____

_____

_____

_____

_____

_____

_____

_____

BIBLIOGRAPHY

Canadian Paediatric Society. (2004, October 9). Canadian Paediatric Society Statement:PP 2004-03. *Maternal depression and child development*, pp. 575–583.

Dunbar, P. L. (1913). *"We Wear the Mask". Lyrics of Lowly Life*. Retrieved from Lit2Go Edition: https://etc.usf.edu/lit2go/187/lyrics-of-lowly-life/3819/we-wear-the-mask/

Janice H. Goodman, P. (2009). Women's attitudes, preferences, and perceived barriers to treatment for perinatal depression. *Birth Issues in Perinatal Care*, 60-69.

Karen Pechman, M. (2014, July 1). *Burke Rehabilitation Hospital*. Retrieved from Montefiore Health System: https://www.burke.org/blog/2014/7/what-you-need-to-know-about-prehabilitation/19

Malcolm A. West, P. E. (2017). Prehabilitation and Nutritional Support to Improve Perioperative Outcomes. *Curr Anesthesiol Rep*, 340-349.

Mayo Clinic Staff. (2018, May 3). *Postpartum Preeclampsia*. Retrieved from Mayo Clinic: https://www.mayoclinic.org/diseases-conditions/postpartum-preeclampsia/symptoms-causes/syc-20376646

Nur, G. D. (2018). Level of Mother-Baby Bonding and Influencing Factors During Pregnancy and Postpartum Period. *Psychiatria Danubina*, 433-440.

Optimizing Postpartum Care. (2018, May).

Pat F. Bass III, M. M. (2018, September 1). *Parental postpartum depression: More than "baby blues"*. Retrieved from Contemporay Pediatrics : http://www.contemporarypediatrics.com/neonatalperinatology/parental-postpartum-depression-more-baby-blues

Pearson, R. (2018, August 6). *The Conversation*. Retrieved from The Conversation: US: https://theconversation.com/mental-health-depression-and-anxiety-in-young-mothers-is-up-by-50-in-a-generation-100914

Peckel, L. (2016, November 21). *Effects of Maternal Pre- and Postpartum Depression on Child's Brain Development*. Retrieved from Neurology Advisor: https://www.neurologyadvisor.com/pediatric-neurology/maternal-pre-and-postpartum-depression-affects-childs-brain-development/article/574413/

Pilyoung Kim, M. B. (2007). Sad Dads: Paternal Postpartum Depression. *Psychiatry*, 36-47.

Psychiatric Rehabilitation. (n.d.). Retrieved 10 29, 2018, from National Center for Biotechnology Information, U.S. National Library of Medicine: https://www.ncbi. nlm.nih.gov/mesh/2009693

World Health Organization. (2018, November 20). *Risk Factors.* Retrieved from World Health Organization: http://www.who.int/topics/risk_factors/en/

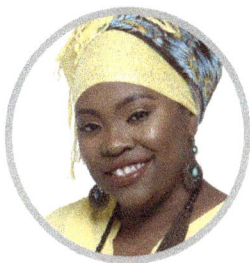

ABOUT THE AUTHOR

Dr. Raushanah Hud-Aleem (a.k.a. Dr. Raushanah) is a bestselling author, speaker, consultant, board-certified general psychiatrist and board-certified child and adolescent psychiatrist. She meets with mothers and their loved ones, one-on-one and in groups, to educate and promote mental health awareness and wellness, while decreasing stigma. She has treated thousands of patients with mental health difficulties.

Dr. Raushanah graduated from Ohio University College of Osteopathic Medicine in 2004. Afterwards, she completed a general psychiatry residency and a child and adolescent psychiatry fellowship at Wright State University Boonshoft School of Medicine, which afforded her the opportunity to train in rural and urban settings. She also trained at a military base where she served active duty members, retirees, and their families.

A former National Health Service Corp member and current member of the American Psychiatric Association, American Academy of Child and Adolescent Psychiatry, and Postpartum Support International. Dr. Raushanah has extensive experience in and fiery passion for community psychiatry and telepsychiatry.

To connect, email her at info@drraushanah.com

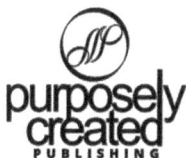

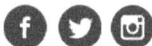